ESSENTIAL GUIDE TO TINEA VERSICOLOR

Understanding, Treating, and Managing Tinea Versicolor: An Essential Guide for Dermatological Wellness

DR. CASEY LOREN

1

DISCLAIMER

This book's content is only meant to be used for general informative purposes. Although the author has taken great care to ensure the content is accurate and thorough, no warranties or assurances on the information's accuracy, correctness, or reliability are provided. It is recommended that readers employ their own judgment and discretion when applying any material found in this book to their particular situation.

The information in this book is not intended to replace professional advice, nor is the author an expert in any of the subjects covered. It is recommended that readers consult with experienced professionals regarding any particular issues or concerns.

Any name that may be mentioned or referred in this book does not imply endorsement, recommendation, or relationship on the part of the author with any person, entity, good, website, or association. These references are made only for informational purposes and are not meant to be taken as recommendations or endorsements.

The information contained in this book may cause readers to suffer loss or damage, for which the author disclaims all obligation and accountability. The only people accountable for the decisions and actions taken by readers using the information presented are themselves.

Any names, characters, companies, locations, activities, occasions, and incidents referenced in this book are either made up or the result of the author's imagination. Any likeness to real people, living or dead, or to real things is entirely coincidental.

This book's content may change at any time, without prior notice, according to the author. The onus is on the reader to verify whether there have been any updates or revisions.

The reader accepts the conditions of this disclaimer by reading this book. Please do not read this book or use its contents if you do not agree to these terms.

Table of Contents

CHAPTER 1

TINEA VERSICOLOR: AN OVERVIEW

Tinea Versicolor: What It Is and How It Works

A common fungal illness of the skin is tinea versicolor, which is sometimes called pityriasis versicolor. An overabundance of the skin-dwelling yeast Malassezia is the root cause of this condition. Patches of discoloured skin, which may be brighter or darker than the rest of the skin, might be a symptom of this illness.

Background and Historical Information

There are historical records that go back to ancient civilizations that mention Tinea versicolor, thus it has been known for ages. Nevertheless, the precise fungus source was not recognised and comprehended until the nineteenth and twentieth centuries. This illness has been extensively investigated and is now curable.

Problems and What Could Go Wrong

An excess of the Malassezia yeast on the skin is the primary reason behind tinea versicolor. Heat and humidity, sebum production, hormonal shifts (during puberty or pregnancy, for example), compromised immunity, and profuse perspiration are all factors that might amplify this overgrowth.

Tinea Versicolor Indicators and Outcomes

Tinea versicolor is characterised by the appearance of brown spots on the skin, most commonly on the upper arms, back, neck, and chest. Mild itching or scaling may accompany these areas, which can be darker or lighter than the surrounding skin.

Methods for Diagnosis

Clinical evaluation and visual skin examination are typically sufficient for the diagnosis of tinea versicolor. The existence of a fungus can be confirmed by a skin scraping or by using a Wood's lamp, a specific type of UV light.

Why Prompt Diagnosis and Treatment Are Crucial

In order to stop the infection from spreading and to lessen the likelihood of a recurrence, tinea versicolor must be treated promptly after diagnosis. Depending on the seriousness of the illness, treatment usually include antifungal drugs, which can be in the form of oral pills, topical creams, or shampoos.

Typical Errors Regarding Tinea Versicolor

It is often believed that tinea versicolor can spread from person to person. The truth is that you can't really catch the disease from someone else until you come into close contact with them.

Effect on Well-Being

Although tinea versicolor is typically not a life-threatening illness, the noticeable symptoms can greatly affect one's standard of living. When the patches are more apparent in the warmer months, some people may feel embarrassed or self-conscious about how their skin looks.

Research on the Causes and Rates of

Fungal infections like tinea versicolor are quite prevalent and can affect anyone of any age or skin type. Adolescents and young adults are more likely to experience it, and it is more common in regions with warm and humid weather.

Research on Tinea Versicolor Has Advanced

More effective therapies for tinea versicolor have been developed as a result of advances in our knowledge of the condition's origins. New therapy options and tactics for preventing recurrence are being explored in ongoing research.

Individuals may take charge of their health and make strides towards a better quality of life by learning about tinea versicolor and its impact, as well as its definition, causes, symptoms, and diagnosis.

CHAPTER 2
DETERMINING THE ROLE OF FUNGI

A Brief Introduction to Malassezia Fungus:

Naturally present on human skin are yeast-like fungus belonging to the genus Malassezia. Although this genus is normally present on the skin, some species can cause infections like tinea versicolor. Fungal infections are prevalent in the scalp, face, and upper trunk because these regions of the skin produce a lot of sebum and are therefore ideal for these lipophilic fungi.

Tinea versicolor and the Function of Malassezia:

Tinea versicolor, often called pityriasis versicolor, is caused by the fungus Malassezia. Discoloured areas, usually lighter or darker than the surrounding skin, are a hallmark of this illness. The characteristic spots on the skin are caused by substances produced by certain species of Malassezia, namely Malassezia globosa and Malassezia furfur.

Various Malassezia Species

Several species of Malassezia have been discovered, including globosa, furfur, sympodialis, restricta, and slooffiae in particular. Different kinds of fungi can cause tinea versicolor in different ways due to differences in biochemical characteristics and pathogenicity.

Malassezia Life Cycle

Malassezia may be either a yeast or a hypha at any point in its life cycle. Yeast cells proliferate mostly on the surface of the skin, where they feed on dead cells and budding off new ones. Malassezia may become pathogenic when subjected to specific environmental factors including elevated humidity and sebum production, which cause the fungus to transform into its hyphal form.

Aspects Influencing the Growth of Malassezia

Malassezia proliferates on the skin depending on a number of variables. A few examples are the following: temperature, humidity, sebum production, skin pH, and immunological reactions of the host. Modifications to these elements can influence the growth and activity of Malassezia in one way or another.

Human Skin Interactions:

Several pathways are involved in the interaction between human skin and Malassezia. of order to survive, it feeds on sebaceous lipids and clings to keratinocytes, the main cells of the epidermis. Its colonisation and survival on the skin surface depend on this contact.

Malassezia Immune Response:

In response to Malassezia, the immune system employs both innate and adaptive pathways. Immune cells such macrophages, dendritic cells, and T lymphocytes are activated when Malassezia antigens are recognised. Tinea versicolor can develop when Malassezia overpopulates a person's skin due to an abnormal immunological response.

Environmental Factors Influencing the Multiplication of Fungi:

The growth of Malassezia fungus is greatly affected by environmental conditions. Their growth is best supported by warm and humid temperatures, while dry and cool climates are less favourable. Tinea versicolor outbreaks might become more common or less severe depending on changes in environmental conditions.

The Relationship Between Malassezia and Additional Skin Disorders

Malassezia is not just associated with tinea versicolor, but with a number of other skin disorders as well. Folliculitis caused by

Malassezia, seborrhoeic dermatitis, and pityriasis folliculorum are all examples of such conditions. A key component in the development of these diseases is the interaction between Malassezia and the microenvironment of the skin.

Looking Ahead for Malassezia Studies

The disease processes, host interactions, and possible treatment targets of Malassezia are the subject of ongoing research. Genomic, proteomic, and immunological advances are clarifying the complexities of skin problems caused by Malassezia and may pave the way for new preventative and therapeutic approaches. Clinicians, microbiologists, and immunologists must work together if we are to make progress in this field.

CHAPTER 3

PRESENTATION OF TINEA VERSICOLOR IN CLINICAL PRACTICE

In most cases, tinea versicolor will manifest with a wide range of skin alterations and lesions. Macules or patches that are either hypopigmented (lighter than the surrounding skin) or hyperpigmented (darker than the surrounding skin) can be found in these areas. They can be circular or oval in shape. The lesions could eventually merge into bigger regions.

Variants with High Pigmentation vs. Low Pigmentation

The lesions caused by tinea versicolor with high pigmentation stand out from the surrounding skin and can be brown, tan, or reddish in colour. On the other hand, hypopigmented patches are lighter in colour and may be slightly pink or whitish.

Body locations Affected by Tinea Versicolor: The groyne, upper arms, neck, and trunk are typical locations where sebum production is strong. Face lesions are more common in young people and teenagers.

It is critical to distinguish tinea versicolor from other skin illnesses such vitiligo, pityriasis rosea, and seborrhoeic dermatitis in order to make an accurate diagnosis. Confirmation of the diagnosis can be achieved through clinical examination, microscopical analysis of skin scrapings, and culture of fungi.

Although most people with tinea versicolor don't feel any symptoms at all, some people may find that the lesions are slightly itchy or burn a little bit, particularly if they're inflamed or irritated.

Factors Influencing Lesion Severity

Some factors can make tinea versicolor lesions worse, including as high temperatures, high humidity, perspiration, and immunosuppression (such as in HIV/AIDS or following organ donation). The severity of a lesion may also be amplified by oily skin and changes in hormone levels.

Tinea versicolor can happen at any age, however it most frequently strikes young adults and teenagers. The presentation of the condition is influenced by gender as well. It seems to be more common in men than in women, which could be because of hormonal variations or the fact that men produce more sebum.

Although tinea versicolor usually shows up as classic lesions, there have been reports of unusual types including folliculocentric, pustular, and erythematous variants. Hyperpigmentation after inflammation or subsequent bacterial infections due to scratching are uncommon complications.

Tinea versicolor can cause visible changes in pigmentation and surface texture, which can have a profound effect on skin colour and texture. In contrast to the smoother but lighter-looking hypopigmented patches, hyperpigmented ones may seem darker and rougher.

Results from the Visual and Dermoscopy Examinations

Tinea versicolor is visually identified by the presence of distinctive round to oval-shaped spots of variable pigmentation. Dermoscopy can clarify the diagnosis of tinea versicolor by revealing the pigmentary changes, follicular plugging, and fine scale that are hallmarks of the condition.

The correct diagnosis and treatment of tinea versicolor depend on a thorough understanding of these clinical signs and traits. Topical and oral antifungal medicine, recurrence prevention strategies, and management of risk factors are the main components of standard treatment.

CHAPTER 4

METHODS FOR DIAGNOSIS

clinical evaluation and patient history:

The first step in doing a clinical assessment is to collect relevant patient information, including symptoms, medical history, and any recent travel or exposure to possible triggers. Scaling, itching, and changes in skin colour, particularly in places that sweat a lot, are symptoms that doctors would look for when diagnosing Tinea Versicolor. Furthermore, they would make note of any prior episodes or treatments, along with any familial history of such skin disorders.

Methods for Conducting a Physical Examination:

Dermatologists search for hypo- or hyperpigmented macules or patches on the skin, usually in places like the neck, back, shoulders, and chest, during a physical examination for the telltale symptoms of Tinea Versicolor. The size, shape, and texture of the lesions, as well as any swelling or scaling that may be present, will be evaluated during the examination.

Diagnostic Instruments in Dermatology

Dermatological instruments, such as dermoscopy or portable magnifying devices, can help to confirm a diagnosis of Tinea Versicolor by revealing minute changes in skin colour and texture. These instruments can make it easier to spot tiny scales or differences in pigmentation than what the human eye can see.

Examination of KOH in the Lab

For the purpose of diagnosing fungus infections such as Tinea Versicolor, a typical laboratory test is the potassium hydroxide (KOH) examination. By dissolving keratin and making any fungal components visible under a microscope, KOH is used to treat a sample of skin scrapings from the afflicted area. The existence of Malassezia yeasts can be confirmed with this test.

Examining Wood Under a Wooden Lamp:

The ultraviolet light emitted by a Wood's lamp can bring attention to Tinea Versicolor and other fungal illnesses. Under the Wood's light, parts that are infected may fluoresce a coral pink or yellow-green colour, which can help with the diagnosis. Nevertheless, further testing may be necessary to corroborate the results using this procedure.

Malassezia Cultivation Methods

In order to determine which species of Malassezia causes Tinea Versicolor, culturing methods include collecting skin samples and cultivating them in a controlled environment. In order to make an informed decision about treatment, culture testing can reveal whether or not the specific strain of fungus is sensitive to antifungal drugs.

Examination of the Structure and Function

Histopathological analysis of skin biopsy samples may be conducted when the diagnosis is not apparent or when additional confirmation is required. As an example, yeast can develop in the stratum corneum of skin, which is a telltale sign of Tinea Versicolor, which can be seen by magnification of tissue sections.

Challenges in Differential Diagnosis

Differential diagnosis can be challenging when dealing with Tinea Versicolor because of its resemblance to other skin disorders. Differentiating Tinea Versicolor from other disorders that look similar requires a thorough evaluation of clinical symptoms, the administration of relevant tests, and consideration of the patient's medical history.

Why a Thorough Assessment is Necessary:

Accurate diagnosis and effective management of Tinea Versicolor require a full evaluation that includes a complete medical history, a physical examination, and the right diagnostic tests. As a result, more specific treatments can be considered when other possible causes of skin abnormalities have been eliminated.

Guidelines and Algorithms for Diagnosis

When diagnosing people who may have Tinea Versicolor, diagnostic algorithms and recommendations give medical professionals with systematic ways to follow. Following these algorithms, which are based on the latest research and dermatological best practices, one may expect a detailed process that includes asking a patient's history, doing a physical examination, and ordering a battery of targeted diagnostic tests.

Healthcare providers can manage Tinea Versicolor with confidence by utilising these diagnostic procedures, which improves patient satisfaction and outcomes.

CHAPTER 5
METHODS OF TREATMENT

Applying Antifungal Agents Topically

The mainstay of Tinea Versicolor treatment is topical antifungal medications. They are effective because they stop the infection-causing fungus from growing. Topical antifungals such as miconazole, terbinafine, ketoconazole, and clotrimazole are commonly utilised. In most cases, a healthcare provider will recommend applying the drug directly to the affected areas once or twice a day for a few weeks.

Antifungal Medications Taken Orally:

Oral antifungal drugs may be used in instances where Tinea Versicolor is extensive or does not react well to topical therapy. Fluconazole and itraconazole are examples of systemic antifungal medicines. Typically, they are taken on a daily basis for a set amount of time, which can be anything from one week to four weeks, based on how bad the illness is.

Therapies Used in Combination:

For more intensive therapy, combination therapies combine topical and oral antifungal medicines. In order to completely eradicate the fungus, this method may be suggested for severe or recurring instances of Tinea Versicolor.

Treatments Sold Commercially

Antifungal shampoos, lotions, or creams with substances like zinc pyrithione or selenium sulphide are the most common over-the-counter options for Tinea Versicolor. Although these products might help with minor infections, it's crucial to see a doctor if the problem persists or is serious.

Natural and Home-Based Solutions:

When dealing with Tinea Versicolor, some people choose to use home remedies or those that are natural. These can be anything from coconut oil and apple cider vinegar to aloe vera and tea tree oil. There is no solid evidence that these treatments can entirely eradicate the fungal infection, but they may alleviate symptoms for some patients.

Practices in Lifestyle and Personal Hygiene:

The best way to keep Tinea Versicolor from coming back is to keep up with your regular hygiene routine. For example, you should take antifungal soap baths often, avoid sweating too much, wear loose-fitting clothes, and stay out of humid places as much as possible.

Possible Negative Reactions to Therapy:

Irritation, itching, redness, or burning at the area of application are common side effects of oral or topical antifungal medicines. Nausea and abdominal pain are among the gastrointestinal side effects that oral antifungals have the potential to induce. Notify your healthcare practitioner right away if you have any negative side effects.

How Long the Treatment Lasts and What Happens Next:

The severity and responsiveness to therapy determine the duration of treatment for Tinea Versicolor. Oral drugs may be taken for 1 to 4 weeks, while topical therapies are often applied for 2 to 4 weeks. In order to track improvement and make any necessary adjustments to treatment, it is essential to schedule follow-up visits with a healthcare professional.

Dealing with Repeated Incidents:

If you suffer from Tinea Versicolor on a regular basis, your doctor may advise you to take antifungal medication as part of a long-term maintenance programme or to avoid getting the condition during peak season. When it comes to controlling recurring infections, it's crucial to identify and treat underlying risk factors like excessive sweating or immune system abnormalities.

New Approaches to Treatment in the Future:

Dermatology and mycology researchers are always looking for innovative ways to treat Tinea Versicolor. Efficacy and recurrence rates can be improved by the introduction of new antifungal drugs, targeted delivery systems, and immunomodulatory therapy. For the most recent information on treatment alternatives, it is important to keep up with credible medical sources that cover new therapies and to talk to healthcare providers.

CHAPTER 6
PREVENTATIVE MEASURES
Proper Skin Care Routines

- **Regular Bathing**: Suggest that people wash their bodies every day with a gentle soap and water mixture to wash away excess sebum and oils that can lead to the development of fungal infections.

- **Improved Drying**: Stress the significance of completely drying the skin, paying specific attention to the groyne, armpits, and spaces in between the toes where moisture tends to accumulate.

The use of clean linens and towels can help stop the spread of fungal infections from one person to another or from one area of the body to another.

- **Stay Away From Sharing Personal Things**: Spread the word about how dangerous it is to share things like combs, shirts, and towels since they might harbour fungus spores.

Things to Think About Regarding the Environment

- **Humidity Control**: It is recommended to maintain controlled indoor humidity levels, as excessive humidity can foster the growth of fungi.
- **Ventilation**: Keep living areas well-ventilated to avoid condensation. If you don't have skin protection, it's not a good idea to spend a long time in a sauna or hot tub, or anywhere else that's humid or moist.

Selecting Apparel and Fabrics

- **Fashionable Materials**: It is advised to wear loose-fitting garments crafted from natural fibres, such as cotton, to enhance air circulation and decrease perspiration buildup. If you want to keep your skin free of fungal infections, it's best to avoid wearing synthetic materials for an extended period of time. These materials trap heat and moisture, which can lead to skin infections.

Food Factors to Think About

In order to prevent fungal infections, it is important to maintain a strong immune system, which can be achieved through a balanced diet that is rich in nutrients.
- **Reduce Consumption of Sugary and Processed Foods**: Make the case that eating too much sugar and processed food can make fungal overgrowth worse.

Steering Clear of Things That Could Set You Off

Stress can lower the immune system's defences and make people more prone to infections, therefore it's important to promote stress-reduction measures.

- **Keeping Perspiring Under Control**: Suggest avoiding activities that cause perspiration under control unless adequate post-exercise hygiene is practiced.

Why Sun Protection Is Crucial

- **Sunscreen Use**: Highlight the significance of utilising sunscreen with a high SPF to shield the skin from damaging UV radiation; sunburns can impair the skin's ability to fight off diseases.

Beginning with Observation and Introspection

- **Skin Checks**: Get people to check their skin on a regular basis so you can catch any changes or anomalies before they get worse.
- **Timely Intervention**: Stress the importance of seeing a doctor right away if you detect any unusual changes to your skin or any symptoms that don't go away.

Education for Families and Communities

Awareness Campaigns: Back local and family-based educational efforts to get the word out about Tinea Versicolor and how to take care of it.

- **urge Open Communication**: Promote open communication within families and communities to address problems, share knowledge, and urge preventive steps.

Travel Precautions

- **Personal Hygiene Essentials**: It is recommended to bring antifungal soaps or wipes along on vacation, particularly to tropical or humid areas where fungal infections are more prevalent.

- **Proper Hygiene Practices While Traveling**: Remind tourists to maintain proper hygiene practices, such as regular bathing, using clean towels, and avoiding sharing personal goods.

Studies on Hazard Avoidance

In order to protect oneself from Tinea Versicolor, it is important to keep oneself informed about the newest research and advice.
- **Talk to Your Doctor**: It is recommended that you talk to your doctor about your specific risk factors and medical history so they can provide you information and recommendations that are tailored to your needs.

Effective prevention of Tinea Versicolor requires a holistic approach that takes into account environmental consciousness, lifestyle choices, personal cleanliness, and proactive healthcare.

CHAPTER 7

MANAGING TINEA VERSICOLOR IN YOUR HOME

Methods for Dealing with Stress for Mental Health

Emotional challenges can arise when living with Tinea Versicolor. Some ways to deal with stress include keeping a positive attitude, taking care of yourself, and reaching out to people you care about or mental health experts when you need help. Additionally, it might be helpful to practice mindfulness, engage in activities that reduce stress, and prioritise overall wellness.

Effect on Mood and Confidence

The apparent changes to the skin caused by Tinea Versicolor can have an effect on self-esteem and body image. Keep in mind that the illness is rather common and poses no health risks. One way to cope with these effects is to work on one's self-image by practicing self-acceptance, making positive affirmations, and putting more emphasis on one's inner qualities than one's outward appearance.

Peer communities and support networks

It might be really helpful to connect with people who can relate to what you're going through. People can obtain emotional support, share tales, and get advice through support networks and online peer communities. A sense of community and shared experiences can have a good effect on health.

Changes to One's Way of Life

Tinea Versicolor can be better managed with some changes to one's way of life. These may involve following a healthcare provider's advice about the use of antifungal medications, maintaining excellent hygiene, not sweating too much, and wearing clothes that allow air to circulate. The health of your skin can also be improved by eating well and keeping stress levels in check.

Skin Concerns and Upkeep

To keep Tinea Versicolor under control, regular visits to a dermatologist are required. The severity of the illness determines the treatment options, which may involve oral drugs, antifungal shampoos, or lotions. Appointments with a dermatologist for follow-up care can help with maintenance and any necessary therapy adjustments.

The Future and Prognosis

In most cases, treatment for Tinea Versicolor works, and many patients even report lasting improvements. Yet, recurrences can happen, particularly in humid areas or when perspiration is at its highest. You may keep a positive mindset in the long run by following your dermatologist's advice, taking good care of your skin, and keeping an eye out for changes.

Dealing with Future Occurrences

Get in touch with a dermatologist right away if your Tinea Versicolor comes back. They are able to evaluate the problem, make therapy adjustments as needed, and offer advice on how to avoid recurrences in the future. Using antifungal creams on a regular basis, staying out of places with high humidity or heat, and taking care of your skin as a whole are all potential strategies.

Patient Testimonials and Accounts

Insights and support can be gained by listening to the stories and experiences of patients living with Tinea Versicolor. It can be encouraging and uplifting to hear about other people's experiences coping, managing recurrences, and maintaining emotional well-being.

Patient Education Materials

You may find a wealth of useful information on Tinea Versicolor in educational resources including trustworthy websites, informative booklets, and online forums. To help people make educated decisions regarding their health, these resources include subjects such as causes, symptoms, treatment options, and self-care suggestions.

Programmes for Raising Awareness and Advocacy

Efforts to raise public knowledge and advocate for Tinea Versicolor are vital. Reducing stigma, increasing knowledge, and encouraging early detection and treatment are the goals of these campaigns. A better informed and supportive community can be yours through participating in advocacy initiatives or lending your support to awareness campaigns.

In order to help people living with Tinea

Versicolor overcome obstacles, get the assistance they need, and be healthy overall, it is important to address all of these elements.

CHAPTER 8

TINEA VERSICOLOR IN CERTAIN GROUPS OF PEOPLE

Sure thing! Regarding Tinea Versicolor in specific populations, here is an exhaustive guide covering all of the points you have brought up:

Paediatric Factors to Consider

Lighter or darker patches on the skin are a common symptom of Tinea Versicolor in youngsters. Because of differences in skin tone and symptoms that are similar to other skin disorders, diagnosing this population can be problematic. Depending on the child's age, skin sensitivity, and other health issues, topical antifungal medications are usually used for treatment.

Tinea Versicolor in the Elderly:

Tinea versicolor can take on a distinct look in the elderly, with darker spots that are harder to treat. Persistent symptoms may be due to a combination of factors, including decreased skin elasticity and compromised immunological function. Antifungal medication side effects in this population must be closely monitored.

Treating Tinea Versicolor During Pregnancy:

Tinea Versicolor therapies may not work as well on pregnant women's skin due to hormonal changes. For the sake of the unborn child's health, topical antifungals are usually better than systemic drugs. Effective management that puts the health of the mother and her unborn child first requires close cooperation between dermatologists and obstetricians.

Immunocompromised People with Tinea Versicolor:

Severe and recurrent Tinea Versicolor infections are more common in people with impaired immune systems, such as those living with HIV/AIDS or on immunosuppressive medication. Antifungal treatment must be continued for longer periods of time and the underlying immunodeficiency must be addressed in order to avoid recurrence.

People Who Lead Active Lives:

Athletes

Tinea Versicolor is more common in athletes and people who lead active lifestyles because of things like perspiration, garment friction, and sharing equipment. Good personal hygiene, the use of antifungal powders or sprays, and the quick treatment of skin lesions are all ways to avoid the spread and recurrence of fungal infections.

Risks in the Workplace:

People may be more likely to get Tinea Versicolor if they work in an environment where they are constantly exposed to water or high humidity. To avoid getting sick on the job, it's important to wear protective gear, practise good hygiene, and treat any changes to your skin right once.

The Importance of Cultural and Ethnic Factors:

Lesion appearance and distribution can vary across ethnicities, making Tinea Versicolor a potentially diverse presentation. The condition's incidence and management can be impacted by cultural traditions, such as skincare regimes and clothing choices. Customised care requires cultural awareness and comprehension.

Predispositions in Heredity:

Tinea Versicolor susceptibility may be influenced by hereditary variables. A person's immune response, skin barrier function, and vulnerability to fungal infections might be affected by specific genetic variants. To learn more about these tendencies and provide more tailored treatment plans, genetic investigations are continuing.

Conditions That Mix with One Another in the Medical Field:

It can be challenging to diagnose and treat tinea versicolor when it occurs alongside other medical issues like eczema, psoriasis, or diabetes. To treat the fungal infection and any underlying medical issues, a thorough evaluation is necessary, and dermatologists and other doctors must work together.

Customised Strategies for Diverse Audiences:

When managing Tinea Versicolor, it is important to take into account the specific traits and requirements of each population. Many factors must be taken into account, such as the patient's age, whether or not the treatment is safe during pregnancy, procedures for patients with impaired immune systems, changes to one's way of life, cultural sensitivity, genetic predispositions, and the treatment of any coexisting medical issues. Optimal results and patient happiness are achieved through customised therapy programmes.

Tinea Versicolor affects a wide variety of people, and healthcare providers can better serve these communities by keeping these nuances in mind.

CHAPTER 9

ALTERNATIVE AND COMPLEMENTARY MEDICINE

Supplements and Herbal Treatments

The field of complementary and alternative medicine frequently investigates herbal supplements and therapies as potential means of controlling tinea versicolor. Herbs with antifungal characteristics, such as aloe vera, tea tree oil, and neem, may be useful in reducing symptoms. Despite their popularity, these cures should only be used after extensive research on their safety and effectiveness has been conducted in conjunction with a healthcare provider.

Conventional Medical Procedures

Some people throughout the world have found success treating tinea versicolor by looking to traditional medical procedures. As an example, fungus infections are commonly treated with herbal remedies and acupuncture in traditional Chinese medicine (TCM). To better manage the disease, it may be beneficial to investigate these methods alongside traditional therapy.

Taking a Holistic View of Skin Health:

Rather of addressing the skin condition in isolation, a holistic approach takes a more comprehensive view of the patient. Along with traditional and alternative medicine, this may necessitate dietary changes, stress management strategies, and adjustments to one's way of life. To supplement conventional therapies for tinea versicolor, holistic techniques can address underlying imbalances and promote general well-being.

Relaxation Methods

When it comes to controlling tinea versicolor, mind-body approaches such as meditation, mindfulness, and relaxation exercises can be quite helpful. Making these changes to your routine may help alleviate stress, which in turn improves your skin's health and reduces the severity of many skin disorders, including fungal infections.

Dietary Supplements & Supplements

When it comes to promoting healthy skin and immunological function, alternative medicine often suggests specific food programmes and nutritional supplements. In cases of tinea versicolor, su

A well-rounded diet high in anti-inflammatory foods and supplements such as probiotics, zinc, and vitamin D may be recommended.

The Advantages of Yoga and Meditation

In addition to their many other health benefits, yoga and meditation may also help keep skin in good condition. When it comes to controlling tinea versicolor, practices like yoga asanas (poses) and pranayama (breathing methods) can be quite helpful. They help reduce stress, promote circulation, and enhance immune function.

Acupressure and Acupuncture

Traditional Chinese medicine practices like acupuncture and acupressure, which include the stimulation of certain areas on the body, may be worth looking into as a possible means of managing tinea versicolor symptoms. Although further studies are required in this field, acupuncture has helped some people, especially when used in conjunction with other treatments.

Clinics Specialising in Integrative Medicine:

Clinics that practise integrative medicine take a more holistic approach to patient care by combining traditional medical practices with alternative and complementary methods. People looking for holistic treatment options for tinea versicolor may find these clinics useful because they may provide services like nutritional counselling, acupuncture, consultations about herbal medicine, and mind-body therapies.

Research on Alternative and Complementary Medicine:

Efficacy and safety of different complementary therapy techniques for tinea versicolor are being studied in ongoing research. When considering the use of complementary therapies as part of a treatment plan, it is crucial to keep up with the most recent research and seek advice from credible sources or healthcare professionals based on evidence.

Use Based on Evidence and Safety Considerations

It is critical to prioritise safety and apply evidence-based practices when contemplating alternative and complementary therapy for tinea versicolor. If you are considering using herbs, supplements, or alternative treatments in addition to standard medical treatments, it is extremely important to talk to a doctor to be sure they are safe, effective, and suitable.

CHAPTER 10

LOOKING AHEAD AND WHERE RESEARCH IS HEADED

New Directions in the Study of Tinea Versicolor

Fungal infections of the skin, caused by species of Malassezia, are known as tinea versicolor. A number of variables, including changes in lifestyle, more humidity, and changing weather patterns, may explain the sharp uptick in its incidence in recent years. To effectively prevent and control these trends, it is essential to understand them.

Diagnostic Technology Advancements

Diagnosing tinea versicolor has become much easier and more accurate thanks to recent developments in diagnostic technology. This disorder can be accurately and non-invasively diagnosed using techniques including reflectance confocal microscopy (RCM), molecular tests, and dermoscopy.

New Potential Therapies and Their Agents

A paradigm shift in the management of tinea versicolor has occurred with the discovery of new therapeutic targets and medicines. Researchers are actively investigating many paths to improve therapy effectiveness and decrease recurrence rates, such as immunomodulatory medicines and antifungal drugs that target specific species of Malassezia.

Approaches to Precision Medicine

Treatments for tinea versicolor can be fine-tuned using precision medicine techniques by taking into account each patient's unique genetic makeup, immunological response, and microbiome. Treatment outcomes and side effects can be optimised with this personalised strategy.

Dermatology and Artificial Intelligence

The use of AI in dermatology has allowed for the automation of image processing, diagnostic support, and tinea versicolor therapy planning. Algorithms powered by artificial intelligence can help dermatologists make more precise diagnosis and choose the best treatments.

Models of Care That Put Patients First

When it comes to managing tinea versicolor, patient-centered care models stress taking a comprehensive approach that takes into account patients' values, preferences, and past experiences. Treatment adherence and results are both improved by these models' emphasis on patient education, psychological support, and shared decision-making.

Implications for Global Health

The health consequences of Tinea versicolor are substantial worldwide, especially in tropical and high-humidity areas. In order to execute focused public health interventions and lessen the disease burden, it is crucial to understand its epidemiology, risk factors, and impact on quality of life.

Ventures in Collaborative Research

Improving our understanding of tinea versicolor and its treatment requires concerted research efforts involving interdisciplinary teams. Innovation, data exchange, and the implementation of research results into clinical practice are all enhanced by collaborations amongst researchers, physicians, industry partners, and patient advocacy organisations.

Policy and Regulatory Factors to Think About Ensuring the accessibility, efficacy, and safety of tinea versicolor treatments is heavily influenced by regulatory and legislative factors. Policymakers deal with problems including healthcare affordability, insurance coverage, and delivery, while regulatory organisations manage things like drug approvals, quality standards, and post-marketing surveillance.

Important Obstacles and Opportunities in the Treatment of Tinea Versicolor

Disparities in healthcare access, high recurrence rates, and a lack of treatment alternatives for resistant tinea versicolor cases are major obstacles to its management. Overcoming these hurdles and improving patient outcomes is possible through collaborative efforts, new technologies, and continuing research.

By delving into these potential avenues for further study, we can improve our knowledge of tinea versicolor and develop better methods for preventing, diagnosing, and treating the condition, all with an eye towards improving patient and world health.